Acne-Free Skin

Simple Proven Solution To Cure Acne Forever and Live Acne-Free, Discover Powerful Secrets to Acne Freedom

Introduction

I want to thank you and congratulate you for downloading the book, *"Acne-Free Skin: Simple Proven Solution To Cure Acne Forever and Live Acne-Free, Discover Powerful Secrets to Acne Freedom"*.

This book contains proven steps and strategies on how to cure acne naturally. Most commercial acne treatments are very expensive and may be too harsh on the skin. There are several natural remedies that you can use to treat acne and prevent it from recurring. These are safe and very effective. These not only treat skin but leave it healthier and looking better, too.

Read on and find out how.

Thanks again for downloading this book, I hope you enjoy it!

Table of Contents

Chapter 1: Learning About Acne

Pimples, zit, acne – these are just some of the names for a really frustrating skin problem. It affects people of all ages, mostly teenagers. Acne can get really frustrating because it keeps coming back. In desperation, some people would resort to popping the zits, hoping it will shrink and eventually go away. Some use harsh soaps or very expensive products to try to get rid of them.

The truth is most of the acne "treatments" mentioned do not really work. Some of them can worsen the problem, such as by causing the pimples to pop. To truly solve this persistent skin problem, a better understanding of the skin and its structure is essential. A good understanding of how acne develops is also important.

The skin

The skin is the single largest organ in the body. It covers the entire body from head to foot. The structure is basically the same, but varies on some points depending on where it is located. For example, no matter where in the body, the skin is composed of 3 layers: the epidermis, dermis and the hypodermis. However, the thickness and distribution of structures within these layers vary cross the body. The epidermis is thicker in the palms and soles of the feet and thinnest over the lips. More sweat glands are present in the armpits and more oil glands are present in the face. Also, there are more follicles in the facial area, as wells as the upper back. These variations are necessary in order for the skin to carry out its function over that specific body area. This is also why acne does not develop all over the body. It only develops in certain areas.

The skin over the face, chest and upper back have relatively oil and sweat glands. These areas are most prone to develop acne because of the abundance of these structures. Also, the pores over these places are often large and can get easily get clogged, causing acne to develop.

Acne and the skin

Acne develops when the pores of the skin get clogged and infected. The clogging comes from oil and dirt. The infection can come from the natural bacterial flora on the skin or from the environment.

The oil glands (called sebaceous glands) in the skin produce lots of oil. This erodes the skin cells lining the pores. Together, they form plugs that can cause blockage of the follicles. Blocked follicles close to the skin surface bulge outward, forming a whitehead. Plugs that form at the top of the follicle react with the air, and become a blackhead.

Bacteria normally residing in the skin's surface are generally harmless, but when it finds its way into the oil-dead skin cell plug, it rapidly multiplies and becomes a problem. It can cause infection within the pores, which worsens acne. Pus forms within the clogged pores and develops into nodules, spots and cysts.

Too much oil production is often considered as the most likely cause of acne because it invites a series of reactions that can lead to acne formation. There are several factors that affect oil production. One is hormones. Androgens increase during puberty and lasts until early adulthood. This is why teenagers and young adults experience the worst cases of acne. These hormones stimulate the sebaceous glands to increase its rate of oil production.

Dry skin is also one trigger for increased oil production. When the skin is dry, it is prone to damage, aging and bacterial overgrowth. In response, the skin increases its oil production in order to provide a good cover to protect the skin. The oil glands over compensate in an attempt to reduce skin dryness. This is why dry skin is also prone to breakouts.

Acne Myths

Common misconceptions hinder effective acne prevention and treatment. It is important to understand the real reasons why acne develops in order to effectively treat and prevent it from recurring.

The most common myth is that acne is caused by dirty skin. This is why people would wash their faces too often using harsh chemicals in an attempt to keep the skin clean at all times. Unfortunately, this practice actually worsens acne. Excessive washing and the use of harsh chemicals strip off the natural oily protective layer of the skin. This will trigger increased oil production and leave the skin prone to develop acne.

What one eats does not affect the oiliness or dryness of the skin. People often associate eating greasy foods and chocolate with acne breakouts, but studies have proven that this is not the case. These foods do not directly cause acne breakouts.

Why treat acne?

Acne is not just unsightly; it can also increase the skin's risk for other, more serious skin conditions. Affected skin areas can develop deep scarring. Acne can also increase the risk for secondary skin infections. Damaged skin is less able to protect itself from bacteria and fungi, making it more vulnerable.

Hence, acne develops in skin that either too dry or too oily. The key to acne treatment and prevention is to promote better skin health. This means using mild skin products that do not promote skin dryness or oiliness while providing direct treatment on acne.

One good way to ensure this is by using natural skin treatments to treat acne.

Chapter 2: Acne Home Remedies

There are lots of expensive skin products and skin treatments that promise to treat acne, but most of these do not work. Most of them are too harsh that they leave the skin even more prone to breakouts. There actually a lot of mild yet effective (not to mention very inexpensive) ways that can treat acne. Most of these are naturally found in the home-the kitchen cupboard to be more precise. Here are some of the most effective ones:

Steam

Steam therapy may sound a bit too fancy but is actually very simple. Skin clinics would charge a few bucks for this. Save a lot by doing this right in the comfort of the home.

Steam works in several ways. The hot air opens the pores, loosening the oil-dirt-dead skin cell plug. Clearing the pores helps the skin to start to heal itself and heal acne.

The heat can also help in discouraging bacterial growth that can otherwise worsen acne. This, plus the addition of some other antibacterial agents such as garlic can further discourage infections in the clogged pores.

There are home facial steams available. The price ranges from a few dollars to hundreds. All of them work the same way.

Make a homemade facial steam by boiling a pot of water. Transfer the water to a large bowl. Lean over the steam, get a towel and create a makeshift tent over the head. Allow the steam to cover the face for a few minutes, about 10-15. Wash the face with mild soap and water afterwards. Pat dry and apply skin-friendly moisturizer. Do this at least once a day, even if there is no present acne breakout.

Apple cider vinegar

Apple cider vinegar is a very effective natural acne treatment. It contains mild acid that helps to kill any bacteria on the skin that worsen acne. It helps to balance the skin pH to discourage any bacterial overgrowth.

Aside from the antibacterial effects, apple cider vinegar also works as an astringent. It dries up the excess oil on the skin, reducing the development of oil plugs. Be careful not to use too much or too often as it can lead to skin dryness that will worsen acne. For best results, use apple cider vinegar diluted.

A few teaspoons can be added to water and used to wash the face. It can also be diluted and used to soak cotton balls. Apply it directly on the pimples and leave it on the skin for a minimum of 10 minutes. It can be left on the skin overnight. Rinse well afterwards and apply moisturizer.

Sodium Bicarbonate (Baking Soda)

This is one of the oldest effective home acne remedies. Its mild antiseptic properties help reduce the bacteria that worsen breakouts. It also dries up the excess oil on the skin surface. It works by exfoliating the skin through microdermabrasion, sloughing off dead skin cells and removing deep-seated dirt and oils.

Make a mask or facial scrub by mixing water and baking soda. Combine the 2 to make a sticky paste. Use this to wash the entire face or dab small amounts on problem areas. Leave it on the skin for 15 to 20 minutes then rinse well with warm water. Pat dry with a soft washcloth and moisturize.

Egg whites

Egg whites are rich in vitamins and proteins that help treat acne and promote skin healing. Vitamins help in reducing the inflammation on the affected areas. These also help to reduce breakouts. Proteins help in rebuilding skin cells over the scars and replacing the sloughed off dead skin cells. The proteins also help in absorbing excess oil to reduce clogging and food that serve as bacterial nourishment.

This remedy is very easy to prepare and apply. Separate the whites from the yolks of about 3 medium-sized eggs. Get a fork or wire whisk and whip the eggs until they turn frothy. This will break up the surface tension and will make the whites easier to apply on the skin. Set aside for a few minutes. Dip the fingertips on the egg whites and apply all over the face. Give more attention to the affected areas. Keep applying until about 3 to 4 layers of egg whites coat the face. Leave the mask on for 20 minutes or so. Rinse well with warm water and pat dry the skin with a soft towel or washcloth. Apply moisturizer afterwards.

Oatmeal

Oatmeal can work both internally and externally. Eating oats every day helps in keeping better health and balance in the body. It can also help in reducing any inflammatory conditions inside the body that can affect skin health. As a result, oil production returns to normal and reduce breakouts.

Externally, oatmeal can be made into a mask. It reduces inflammation of the affected skin areas. It also reduces the redness that often accompanies a bad breakout. Oatmeal mask can also help absorb excess oil on the skin surface.

Oatmeal is soaked in warm water to form a paste. Or it can be cooked to a pasty consistency. Some opt to add a few teaspoons of honey to amp the acne-busting properties. Let the oatmeal cool to a comfortable temperature before applying all over the face. Allow the oatmeal mask to set and leave it on for 20 to 30 minutes. Rinse well with warm water. Dry the skin gently with a soft towel.

Sugar

The natural grittiness of sugar particles is a good way to gently exfoliate the face. It helps to remove accumulated oil and dirt, as well as dead skin cells from the skin surface and from the pores. Sugar can be added to plain water, olive oil or honey.

One good recipe to try is mixing equal amounts of white and brown sugar with a few tablespoon of coarse sea salt. Add enough olive oil (honey or water) to wet the sugars and salt. Do not add too much that the granules dissolve. Use as facial scrub. Gently exfoliate the skin, especially over the affected areas. Rinse well with water then pat dry. Apply moisturizer.

Do this regularly or once daily. Avoid rubbing too hard. This can lead to scratching the delicate facial skin. it can also worsen scarring.

Milk or Yogurt

Dairy products are often linked to acne breakouts. There is still ongoing debate whether milk and dairy products do trigger acne or not. Some suggest that the hormones in the milk (from hormones given to cows to improve milk production) are what cause the problem. However, more people attest that using milk on the skin promotes better health. Queen Cleopatra of Ancient Egypt was known to take frequent milk baths, and she was said to be the most beautiful woman in her time. That should be enough proof.

Yogurt is also good for the skin. When eaten, it helps to regulate bacterial colony in the intestines. Doing so helps to remove toxins from blood and from all other organs, including the skin. This way, skin health s restored, reducing breakouts. Yogurt can be use directly on the sin. The probiotics content helps in controlling bacterial populations to reduce acne. It promotes skin pH balance that discourages bacteria. The fat in yogurt helps in providing skin moisture and regulates oil production.

Apply milk or yogurt directly on the affected areas. Apply a few layers on the skin until a thick mask is created. Let it set and leave it on the skin for 10 to 15 minutes. Rinse well with water.

Honey

Honey has mild antimicrobial properties. It can help treat infected acne. It also reduces bacterial overgrowth in the skin surface that worsens or promotes breakouts.

Aside from this, honey is also a good anti-inflammatory agent. It reduces the swelling over the pimples and the redness of the surrounding skin. It is so effective that dabbing a small amount of honey on the affected area and leaving it overnight results in better skin appearance in the morning.

Honey also attracts moisture and keeps it within the skin structure. This property makes it a very effective natural moisturizer. Honey on the skin helps keep it plumper, softer, and more supple. All these effects help keep the skin healthy and well nourished, effectively preventing future breakouts.

Honey is often used in combination with other acne treatments. It is added to natural scrubs and masks. Spices and herbs are also added to help boost the effectiveness.

Try using cinnamon and honey mix. Mix 2 tablespoon of honey with 1 teaspoon of cinnamon. Blend thoroughly until the mix resembles a thick paste. Rinse the face and pat dry before applying the honey mix. Use it as a facial mask and apply all over the face. It can also be used for spot treatment by dabbing small amounts on individual pimples. Leave it on the face for 10 to 15 minutes. Rinse well with water and pat dry.

Chapter 3: Acne Herbal Treatments

Nature is abundant in herbs and spices that help treat acne and other skin problems. These herbs and spices are all natural, safe and effective to use on the skin. Use these to clear the skin and keep it healthy, glowing and blemish-free.

Tea tree oil

Tea tree oil is one of the most popular essential oils used for skin treatments. It is one of the most effective and widely used herbal remedy for acne. The oil cuts through the skin oils that clog the pores. This way, it breaks up the plug, making it easier to remove and unclog the pores. Its antibacterial properties kill any bacteria within the pores that can worsen the skin problem.

Take note that tea tree oil is always used on the skin and not to be ingested internally. Before using it on the skin, dilute it with clean water.

Wash and gently dry the face before applying diluted tea tree oil. Dip a Q-tip to diluted oil and apply directly on the affected skin areas. If the skin is extra sensitive, use aloe vera gel for dilution instead of using water. The gel soothes in the inflamed and irritated skin during treatment.

Garlic

Garlic is very popular for its antibacterial properties. It is a good herbal acne remedy because it effectively kills acne-causing bacteria without any negative side effects.

It can be used internally or externally. Eating garlic helps to improve overall health, which would lead to better skin circulation and health. Blemishes clear up from within. Garlic can also be used on the skin. just remember to dilute the juice first before using. Mash up a few cloves of garlic or squeeze the juice out and add a small amount of clean water. Apply it over the acne areas with a Q-tip.

Cinnamon

Cinnamon has a mild antimicrobial effect. It helps to fight off any infections that worsen skin problems. This is often used in combination with honeyfor a potent bacteria-fighting effect.

Mint

The menthol in mint works to soothe inflamed and irritated skin. It also helps to reduce pain that often accompanies a serious breakout. It does not directly treat acne. It only reduces some of the accompanying symptoms such as pain, redness and inflammation.

Crush a handful or so of mint leaves. Rub it all over a previously washed face. Allow the face to absorb the mint juice. Rinse well after 5 to 10 minutes, using cold water.

The skin would look fresher after use. Puffiness and redness is significantly reduced. Plus, there is the cooling effect that refreshes the entire face.

Aloe vera

The gel from the aloe vera leaves also has a cooling, refreshing and soothing effect. It relieves skin inflammation and pain that comes with acne. Aside from this, aloe vera is also a good skin cleanser. It can also fight off infections and help the skin recover from acne.

Using aloe vera is very easy. Break off a leaf and gently press on it to release more of the gel. Rub the gel directly onto the affected area in a circular motion. Leave it for a few minutes before rinsing thoroughly with cool water.

Neem

Neem is more popular in Ayurvedic traditional healing methods. It has potent anti-viral, anti-fungal and anti-bacterial properties. It helps to reduce infections that worsen acne. It is also a good skin detoxifier that helps clear the skin from dirt and toxins. By doing so, skin health is improved, helping the skin to recover from acne better and faster. It also supports the immune system, helping the skin fight of infections better, reducing the severity of breakouts.

Fresh or dried leaves can be used. Crush the leaves and make a paste by mixing it with clean water. Apply on the forehead, chin and cheeks.

Milk thistle and Dandelion

Drinking dandelion or milk thistle tea can detoxify the body. Removing toxins from within helps promote better skin health. It also helps to clear skin blemishes by promoting better blood flow and waste/toxin removal. Tincture of dandelion or milk thistle is added to hot water to make a tea. About 30 drops of each or combination of both herbs is used. Drink the tea 3 times a day. This can also be used directly on pimples. Dip a cotton ball or Q tip on chilled tea and rub over the affected areas.

Olive Leaf Extract

Extract from the leaves of *Olea europaea* is a known herbal remedy for skin conditions. It has been used for such as very long time, as far back as the Ancient Greece.

Olive leaf extract contains compounds that have antimicrobial and antioxidant properties. When used topically, it can reduce microbial overgrowth that promotes breakouts.

The extract can also be used internally. Drinking it promotes internal detoxification. Clearing the blood of toxins and wastes helps to promote better skin health.

It also contains compounds that help to restore hormonal balance. As has been previously mentioned, hormones play a major role on the activity of the sebaceous glands. Olive leaf extract helps to regulate androgens in the body, restoring it to normal levels.

Burdock

The extract is taken from the root of the Burdock plant. It has long been used in traditional medicine for treating skin problems, including acne.

The extract is full of compounds that have very potent antibacterial and anti-inflammatory properties. It specifically kills bacteria linked to acne formation such as *Propionibacterium*. Cysts and nodules in severe forms of acne is visibly reduced after application of burdock root extract.

Lavender Oil

Lavender is known for its very effective antiviral, analgesic and antibacterial properties. It fights bacteria that cause acne. The oil easily penetrates deep into the skin layers to soothe inflammation, irritation, redness and pain associated with breakouts. It also promotes growth of new skin cells to push off dead ones on the skin surface.

The oil is applied directly on the affected areas but should be diluted first. Lavender oil is very strong and may cause skin irritation. Grape seed oil can be used for dilution, to enhance its acne-busting properties.

Chapter 4: Acne Natural Remedies

Some foods can be used to treat acne, too. These foods contain compounds, minerals and vitamins that help the skin heal, fight off bacteria and reduce inflammation. These everyday foods can be used topically (applied on the skin).

Lemon

Juice from lemon is rich in vitamin C. It helps to promote younger-looking, supple and healthy skin. This is good to use on all the different skin types- from dry to oily skin.

Lemon juice also contains citric acid that helps in exfoliating the skin. it gently loosens dead skin cells on the skin surface. This way, dead cells are removed to allow the new skin cells underneath to emerge. Blemishes and scarring are reduced this way. Also, by promoting cell turnover, the skin is able to heal itself from an acne breakout.

Acids from the juice have astringent properties. It helps to reduce the oil production. This will dry out the pimples and speed up healing.

The same acids also help to whiten the skin. Scars left by bouts of acne lightens, which improves the appearance of the skin.

When using lemon juice o the skin, avoid getting it exposed to the sun. The acids leave the skin extra sensitive to sunlight. It becomes more prone to sunburns and damage.

Dab a cotton ball or Q-tip in freshly squeezed lemon juice. Apply it directly on the affected areas for spot treatment. If a stinging sensation is felt, try to add yogurt to the juice for a soothing effect. Rinse well after 15 minutes and pat dry. Apply moisturizers.

Orange

Oranges can help refresh and rejuvenate the skin. Just like lemon juice, orange juice has citric acids and vitamin C that improve skin health. It also has very potent astringent properties to reduce oil production. Orange helps to promote new skin cell growth to treat acne and promote skin healing.

The peel is used in treating acne problems. The orange peel is ground or pounded to bring out the oils. Add a small amount of water while the peel is pounded. Add slowly at a few drops at a time. Keep grinding or pounding to achieve a paste-like consistency. Apply the paste all over the face (as a face mask) or on affected areas (as spot treatment). Keep on the face for 20 to 25 minutes. Rinse with ample amounts of water. Dry the face gently then apply moisturizer.

Papaya

Raw papaya fruit helps to remove dead skin cells that can combine with oil and cause clogged pores and acne. It also removes excess oils on the skin surface. Papain, an enzyme in papaya, also reduces skin inflammation that promotes acne and prevents pus formation within clogged pores.

To use, mash the fruit until it is smooth enough to apply over the face. Leave it for 15 to 120 minutes before rinsing well with ample amounts of water. The skin is left smooth and soft. If the skin tends to dry after treatment, apply additional moisturizers.

Strawberries

Strawberries are naturally high in salicylic acid. This acid is integral in the acne treatment products. It works by promoting epidermal shedding. That is, it promotes the removal of dead epidermal (surface) cells. By doing so, skin turnover and renewal is promoted, speeding up haling and recover from acne.

It can be used alone as a mask or combined with honey. The antibacterial and anti-inflammatory effects of honey add to the effectiveness of strawberry for acne treatment.

To use, mash fresh strawberries, about 3 pieces. Keep mashing until a smooth and even consistency is achieved, but not too runny and watery. Add 2 teaspoon honey and mix them well. Apply on the face as a mask and leave for about 20 minutes. Rinse well with ample amounts of warm water. Dry gently and thoroughly. Apply moisturizers if the skin feels dry and tight. Do this at least twice a week.

Banana

Banana peel contains a potent antioxidant compound called lutein. It works by reducing the inflammation of acne-affected skin. It also stimulates the growth of new skin cells.

Using this to treat acne is very easy. Just remove the banana peel and rub the inside all over the affected areas. Use a circular motion while rubbing the peel. After rubbing all over the face, leave it to allow the compounds to work on the skin. Rinse well after 30 minutes.

Conclusion

Thank you again for downloading this book!

I hope this book was able to help you to heal acne naturally, safely and fast.

The next step is to start rummaging through the kitchen for these remedies and start treating acne. Do not wait any longer because the answer to your acne woes is right there in front of you. Use them now and enjoy better looking skin.

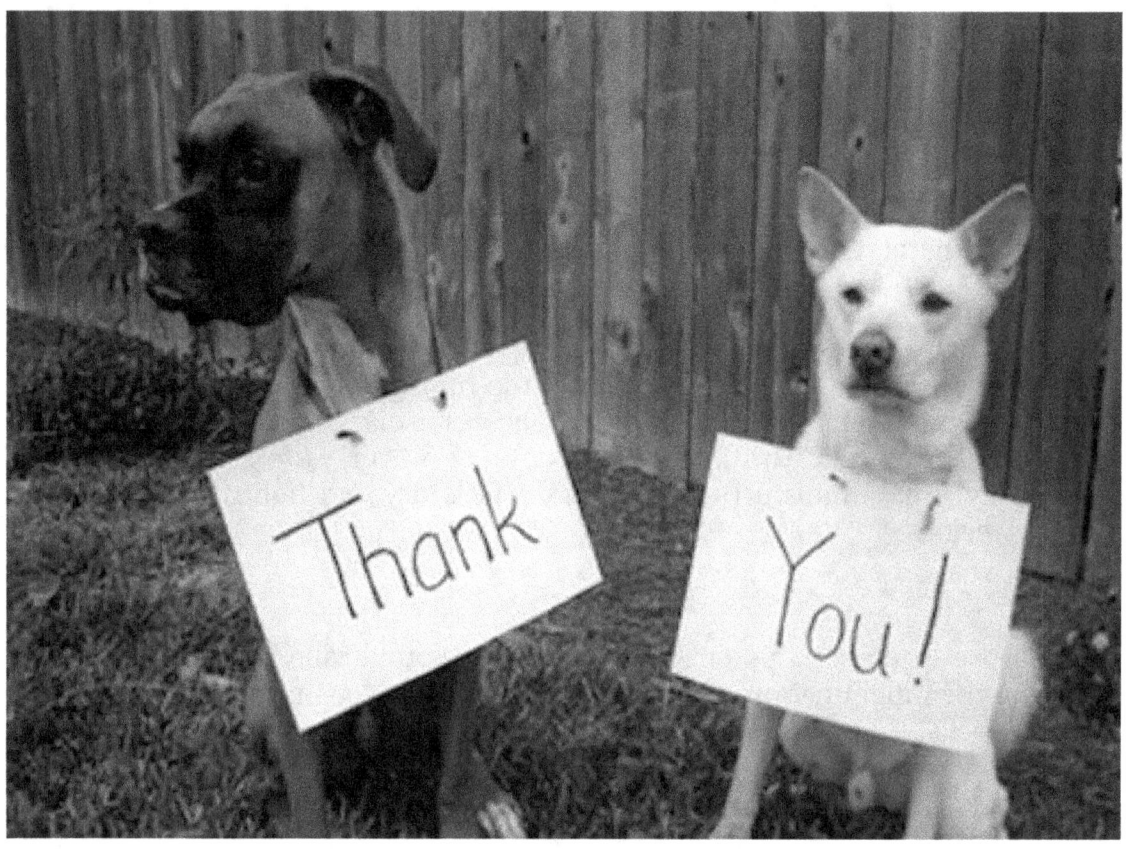

Finally, if you enjoyed this book, then I'd like to ask you for a favor, would you be kind enough to leave a review for this book on Amazon? It'd be greatly appreciated!

Thank you and good luck!

Check Out My Other Books

Below you'll find some of my other popular books that are popular on Amazon and Kindle as well. Simply click on the links below to check them out. Alternatively, you can visit my author page on Amazon to see other work done by me.

Diabetes Solution: Diabetes Guide on How to Incorporate Diabetes Diet and Nutrition Plan for a Diabetes Free Lifestyle

http://www.amazon.com/dp/B00O97FET2

The Blind Truth of Addiction in Society: Drug Addiction Caused by Unemployment, Lack of Education, and Poverty

http://www.amazon.com/dp/B00PDVUKNI

The True Jesus Speaks Out: The Biblical Secrets Revealed, Jesus Was Man Or Was Jesus God?

http://www.amazon.com/dp/B00O349P2I

The Ultimate Guide To Stress Free Parenting: How To become Stress Free Using Stress Free Management Skills.

http://www.amazon.com/dp/B00NZI9XHU

If the links do not work, for whatever reason, you can simply search for these titles on the Amazon website to find them.

Also add me to Facebook so we can chat some:

http://www.facebook.com/talal.sobhey

"This page [is] intentionally left blank."

"**This page** [is] **intentionally left blank**."

"This page [is] intentionally left blank."

"This page [is] intentionally left blank."

"This page [is] intentionally left blank."

"This page [is] intentionally left blank."

"This page [is] intentionally left blank."

"**This page** [is] **intentionally left blank**."

"**This page** [is] **intentionally left blank**."